Inspired by
HULDA REGEHR CLARK

THE CURE FOR ALL DISEASES COOKBOOK

HEALING RECIPES INSPIRED BY DR. HULDA CLARK'S NATURAL CURE FOR ALL DISEASES

STEVEN WIRT

BONUS INSIDE

Table Of Contents

Introduction: What If the Cure Has Been in Your Kitchen All Along?   4
Chapter 1: The Root of All Disease   9
    Parasites, Toxins, and Pollution   9
    The Role of Nutrition in Healing   14
Chapter 2: The Clark Protocol Overview   17
    Herbal Cleanses: Liver, Kidney, and Parasite   18
    The Zapper: Theory and Construction   21
    Diet as Defense: Food as Medicine   23
Chapter 3: The Parasite-Free Pantry   26
    Garlic & Clove Detox Broth   26
    Black Walnut Green Smoothie   27
    Spiced Pumpkin Seed Pesto   28
    Wormwood Tea Elixir   29
    Ginger-Cilantro Parasite Cleanse Soup   30
    Raw Garlic & Olive Tapenade   31
    Clove-Infused Detox Rice   32
    Turmeric-Parsley Detox Tonic   33
    Raw Papaya Anti-Parasite Salad   34
    Anti-Parasitic Spicy Carrot Juice   35
    Pumpkin Seed Snack Mix   36
    Cabbage & Garlic Stir-Fry   37
    Anti-Parasitic Golden Milk   38
    Zucchini & Clove Skillet   39
    Parasite-Cleansing Herb Omelet   40
Chapter 4: Liver and Kidney Loving Recipes   41
    Beet & Carrot Liver Flush Juice   41
    Dandelion Greens & Apple Salad   42
    Parsley-Lemon Detox Tea   43
    Turmeric & Ginger Kidney Broth   44
    Watermelon-Cucumber Kidney Flush   45
    Celery & Apple Juice for Kidneys   46
    Cilantro-Pumpkin Seed Liver Salad   47
    Ingredients (Serves 2):   47
    Kidney Tea Blend   48
    Bitter Greens Liver Bowl   49
    Golden Kidney & Liver Soup   50
    Cucumber-Mint Detox Water   51
    Milk Thistle Smoothie   52

Liver-Loving Sweet Potato Mash	53
Herbal Kidney Detox Infusion	54
Lemon-Olive Oil Liver Shot	55

Chapter 5: Heavy Metal Detox Dishes — 56

Cilantro-Lime Quinoa Bowl	56
Chlorella Green Detox Smoothie	57
Garlic & Broccoli Stir-Fry	58
Cilantro-Pumpkin Seed Pesto Pasta	59
Seaweed & Avocado Wraps	60
Brazil Nut & Spinach Salad	61
Cilantro Detox Dressing	62
Sweet Potato & Parsley Mash	63
Spirulina Detox Shot	64
Bok Choy & Garlic Stir Fry	65
Detox Lentil & Cilantro Soup	66
Lemon-Ginger Detox Water	67
Chlorella Energy Balls	68
Heavy Metal Detox Soup	69
Cilantro & Green Apple Juice	70

Chapter 6: Immune-Strengthening Meals — 71

Immunity Boosting Garlic & Turmeric Soup	71
Ginger-Miso Immunity Broth	73
Vitamin C Super Smoothie	74
Immune Greens Stir-Fry	75
Zinc-Packed Pumpkin Seed Porridge	76
Citrus-Garlic Immunity Shot	77
Fermented Veggie Bowl	78
Reishi Mushroom Tea	79
Immunity Garden Salad	80
Garlic-Lemon Roasted Cauliflower	81
Turmeric Lentil Stew	82
Green Immunity Juice	83
Sesame-Garlic Bok Choy	84
Yogurt-Parfait Power Cup	85
Spiced Golden Milk Latte	86

Chapter 7: Alkalizing and Anti-Mold Recipes — 87

Alkaline Green Juice	87
Avocado-Cucumber Soup (Raw & Chilled)	88
Quinoa Detox Bowl	89
Steamed Broccoli with Garlic-Oregano Oil	90
Zucchini Noodles with Basil-Pumpkin Seed Pesto	91

Anti-Mold Cabbage Slaw	92
Lemon-Thyme Roasted Carrots	93
Alkaline Seed Crackers	94
Fennel & Arugula Detox Salad	95
Turmeric-Almond Milk Tonic	96
Mold-Free Coconut Yogurt Parfait	97
Cucumber-Mint Detox Water	98
Ginger-Lime Marinated Mushrooms	99
Baked Lemon-Cilantro Cauliflower Rice	100
Mold-Free Alkaline Veggie Stir-Fry	101
Bonus Chapter : 30 Day Meal Plan	**102**
Week 1	102
Week 2	104
Week 3	105
Week 4	107
Conclusion: Returning to Nature, Reclaiming Your Health	**110**

Introduction: What If the Cure Has Been in Your Kitchen All Along?

You're here because something doesn't feel right.

Maybe you've been living with chronic fatigue, digestive issues, foggy thinking, stubborn skin conditions, or an endless carousel of medical appointments that never seem to resolve the root of your health problems. Maybe you've sensed, deep down, that something in your body is off—and that the answers you've been given are just pieces of a much larger, missing puzzle.

This book was written for you.

Welcome to THE CURE FOR ALL DISEASES COOKBOOK—a bold, practical, and transformative guide inspired by the groundbreaking work of Dr. Hulda Regehr Clark. Her message was simple, **yet revolutionary**: all diseases have a cause, and once the cause is known, the cure becomes not only possible—but often shockingly simple.

If you've ever felt overwhelmed by conflicting advice, worried about hidden toxins in your food, or frustrated by treatments that only manage symptoms rather than eliminate them—this book will feel like a breath of fresh air. Because here, we don't treat disease as a mystery. We treat it as a message—one that can be decoded and answered using the wisdom of nature, the power of clean food, and the healing systems your body already knows how to use.

This Is Not Just a Cookbook. This Is a Healing Manual.

Unlike other cookbooks, The Cure for All Diseases Cookbook isn't about calories, food trends, or fad diets. It is about healing at the cellular level—cleansing the body from parasites, toxins, mold, heavy metals, and chemical residues that silently sabotage your health.

This book serves as your step-by-step guide to achieving that goal. Rooted in Dr. Clark's time-tested protocols, **each chapter is carefully designed to help you:**

- Eliminate the hidden parasites and pathogens living in your gut and organs
- Detoxify the liver and kidneys, your body's vital filtration systems
- Eliminate toxic heavy metals such as mercury, aluminum, and lead from your body
- Naturally boost your immune system with foods packed with antiviral, antifungal, and parasite-fighting nutrients
- Alkalize your body, restoring internal pH balance to fight off disease
- Avoid mold and chemical residues that poison the blood and weaken your energy

And the best part? It's all done with food.

The recipes in this book are powerful, delicious, and intentionally crafted using only the cleanest ingredients. They follow the principles of Dr. Clark's parasite cleanse, liver detox, kidney support, and anti-mold protocol—so every bite you take becomes an act of healing.

You'll also find detailed guidance on how to stock your pantry, prepare meals safely, and avoid the common food traps that contribute to disease, fatigue, and aging.

If You've Tried Everything and Nothing Has Worked—This Is Your Turning Point

You may have already tried "**clean eating**." You may have already visited countless specialists. You may be taking medications or supplements that were supposed to work—but haven't.

But here's what most protocols miss: disease is not random. It has a cause. And that cause is often overlooked in modern medicine.

Dr. Clark discovered that hidden parasites, molds, solvents, and industrial toxins accumulate in our bodies over time—through food, water, air, and everyday products. These invaders disrupt our natural systems, overload the liver, and weaken the immune response. But when we remove the invaders and support the body's natural detoxification, healing begins.

That's what this book is about. It's not theory—it's actionable, life-restoring nutrition that works with your body, not against it.

The Real Cure Is Simpler Than You've Been Led to Believe

We've been taught that the cure for disease is hidden in a laboratory. That healing comes in the form of pills, surgeries, and complicated technologies. **But what if there's more to the story than we've been told?**

What if the real cure is sitting in your kitchen right now?

What if garlic, ginger, wild herbs, leafy greens, ancient grains, mineral-rich broths, **and wild-caught proteins hold the keys to the healing you've been searching for?**

What if you didn't need more diagnoses—but less toxicity?

What if your body, once unburdened, knows exactly how to repair itself?

This is the truth behind **The Cure for All Diseases Cookbook**. It's not about managing illness. It's about reclaiming wellness.

What You'll Find Inside

- 75+ healing recipes designed for real, restorative change
- A 30-Day meal plan using the entire recipe collection for full-body support
- Guidelines for building a parasite-free, toxin-free pantry
- Recipes made without gluten, refined sugar, mold contaminants, or artificial preservatives
- Insights into how food affects the liver, kidneys, immune system, gut, and brain
- And guidance on how to use food in tandem with Dr. Clark's protocols—including her herbal cleanses and frequency-based zapper device

You Were Meant to Heal

Your body is not broken. It is not deficient in pharmaceuticals. It is designed with intelligence and purpose.

This book is a tool to help you return to that design—to clean out what doesn't belong, nourish what does, and give your body the space it needs to thrive.

You're not just about to read another cookbook. You're about to begin a new relationship with food, with healing, and with the truth.

Let **The Cure for All Diseases Cookbook** be your guide back to the vibrant, disease-free life you deserve.

Because healing doesn't start in a hospital. It starts in your kitchen. **And it starts now.**

Chapter 1: The Root of All Disease

Parasites, Toxins, and Pollution

Modern medicine often seeks to manage symptoms rather than address their underlying cause. **The consequence?** Chronic diseases that linger, resurface, or morph into more serious conditions despite a barrage of pills and procedures. But what if the answer isn't more medical complexity—**but radical simplicity?**

According to Dr. Hulda Regehr Clark, the root cause of virtually all disease—yes, all disease—boils down to a few very manageable culprits: parasites, toxins, and pollution. These silent saboteurs invade the body, disrupt organ function, suppress immunity, and create an internal environment where sickness thrives. The good news is that with knowledge, commitment, and a return to natural foods and remedies, we can reclaim our health.

This chapter explores the foundational philosophy of this cookbook—why disease develops and how nutrition can play a pivotal role in reversing it.

Parasites: The Hidden Intruders

Dr. Clark's groundbreaking research revealed a shocking truth: parasites are far more common in humans than previously thought, and their presence is linked to everything from cancer and diabetes to depression and epilepsy.

Parasites—organisms that live inside a host to survive—can inhabit virtually any part of the body: liver, brain, intestines, even muscles. They are not exclusive to underdeveloped nations or unsanitary environments. In fact, Dr. Clark's studies showed that many North Americans are unknowingly infected due to contaminated food, water, household products, and even cosmetic items.

The most dangerous parasite identified in her work is the human intestinal fluke (**Fasciolopsis buski**), which she associated with a wide variety of degenerative diseases, including cancer. But these organisms don't act alone. For them to trigger a full-blown disease process, certain conditions must be present—most notably, the presence of solvents and toxins in the body.

How Parasites Cause Disease

1. **Organ Invasion**: Parasites can migrate to vital organs, disrupting their function.
2. **Immune Suppression**: Their presence taxes the immune system, making the body more vulnerable to infection and inflammation.
3. **Toxin Production:** Parasites release waste that burdens detox organs like the liver and kidneys.
4. **Chronic Inflammation**: Their lifecycle and movement often trigger inflammatory responses that never fully resolve.

Toxins and Pollution: The Modern Epidemic

If parasites are the soldiers in this war on your health, toxins are chemical weapons. Every day, the average person is exposed to hund' chemicals—from pesticides on produce and heavy metals in tap water to phthalates in cosmetics and volatile organic compounds in cleaning supplies.

Dr. Clark discovered that these substances don't just pass through the body—they accumulate in tissues, disrupt enzymatic processes, and interact synergistically with parasites to ignite disease. A parasite might not cause cancer on its own, but in the presence of isopropyl alcohol (a common solvent), its DNA-damaging potential is amplified exponentially.

Common Toxins Identified by Dr. Clark:

- **Isopropyl Alcohol**: Commonly present in store-bought lotions, mouthwashes, and household cleaning products.
- **Benzene**: Present in soft drinks, processed foods, and some vitamin supplements.
- **Heavy Metals (Lead, Mercury, Aluminum)**: Frequently found in dental fillings, cookware, tap water, and antiperspirants.
- **Food Additives (MSG, Aspartame, Preservatives)**: Widespread in processed and convenience foods.
- **Mold Mycotoxins**: Contaminants found in old grains, nuts, and moldy environments.

The Accumulation Effect

Most people assume the body detoxifies efficiently, but that's not always true. Over time, the accumulation of microscopic doses of toxic substances can weaken the immune system, disrupt hormonal balance, and create a hospitable terrain for parasites and chronic infections.

Pollution of Food and Water: Silent Saboteurs

In her work, Dr. Clark emphasized that clean food and water are the foundation of health. Unfortunately, our modern supply is anything but clean.

Food Pollution

- **Rancid Oils**: Cooking oils like canola or corn become oxidized during processing and disrupt cell membranes.
- **Pesticide Residue**: Found on non-organic fruits, vegetables, and grains.
- **Hormones and Antibiotics**: Present in conventional meat and dairy products.
- **Plasticizers (like BPA)**: Leach from food containers, disrupting endocrine function.
- **Mold Contamination**: Nuts, grains, and breads can be infected with invisible mycotoxins.

Water Pollution

Tap water often contains:

- **Chlorine**: Disrupts gut flora and weakens immunity.
- **Fluoride**: Linked to thyroid dysfunction and neurological impairment.
- **Heavy Metals**: Arsenic, lead, and aluminum are routinely found in municipal water systems.

Even filtered water may not be safe if filters are not maintained properly. According to Dr. Clark, distilled water is the gold standard for daily use, especially during cleansing.

The Role of Nutrition in Healing

Now that we understand the root causes of disease, we can begin to see how food becomes not just a source of fuel—but a source of medicine.

Nutrition has the power to:

- Starve parasites.
- Support detox organs.
- Neutralize toxins.
- Strengthen immune responses.
- Rebuild damaged tissue.

When food is pure, alive, and strategically selected, it becomes a potent force for regeneration.

Nutritional Principles from Dr. Clark's Protocol

1. **Clean and Whole Foods Only**
    - No processed foods.
    - No artificial additives, sweeteners, colors, or preservatives.
    - Choose organic whenever possible to minimize contact with harmful pesticides.
2. **Parasite-Resistant Diet**
    - Garlic, onion, clove, and black walnut inhibit parasite growth.
    - Avoid raw fish, undercooked meats, and unwashed produce.
3. **Support for Detox Pathways**
    - **Liver-loving foods**: beets, dandelion greens, lemons.
    - **Kidney-supportive foods**: parsley, celery, cucumbers.

- **Foods high in sulfur**: such as garlic, cabbage, and broccoli.

4. **Immune Strengthening**
    - Fruits and vegetables packed with antioxidants
    - Fermented foods to support a healthy balance of gut bacteria
    - Zinc, vitamin C, and selenium from whole food sources.

5. **No Aluminum, BPA, or Plastic Leaching**
    - Use glass, stainless steel, and ceramic cookware.
    - Avoid aluminum foil and plastic wrap.

6. **Water as Medicine**
    - Drink only distilled or spring water.
    - Avoid commercial bottled water unless verified BPA-free.

The Synergy of Food and Cleanse

Dr. Clark's herbal parasite cleanse (**black walnut hull, wormwood, and cloves**) is powerful, but its effects are magnified when combined with the right food. Each meal in this cookbook is designed not just to nourish, but to cleanse, regenerate, and empower.

These recipes aim to:

- Starve and eliminate parasites.
- Bind and expel toxins.
- Nourish the liver, kidneys, and immune system.
- Provide anti-inflammatory, alkalizing, and energizing effects.

By following the principles in this book, your kitchen becomes not just a place to cook—but a sacred space of cellular healing.

A Return to Simplicity

Disease is not random. It is not inevitable. And it is not permanent when the true cause is removed. Dr. Hulda Clark's approach restores agency to the individual—empowering you to take health into your own hands.

By eliminating parasites, detoxifying from pollutants, and nourishing the body with healing foods, you begin a journey of true regeneration.

And this book is your roadmap.

In the next chapter, we'll dive deeper into The Clark Protocol—including the precise herbal cleanses and the electrical device known as The Zapper, which together with healing foods form the triad of natural recovery.

But before you go there, take this to heart:

- "True healing can't occur in the same environment that caused your illness. Change the food, clean the water, expel the invaders, and nourish what is left. The body knows what to do."
  — Dr. Hulda Regehr Clark

Chapter 2: The Clark Protocol Overview

Herbal Detoxes: Targeting the Liver, Kidneys, and Parasites — **The Zapper**: Principles and How to Build It — **Nutrition as Protection**: Using Food as Medicine

In Chapter 1, we uncovered the foundational understanding that most diseases stem from just a few core culprits: parasites, toxins, and pollutants. Dr. Hulda Regehr Clark's work showed us that by identifying and removing these hidden root causes, we could reverse even the most advanced illnesses.

But how exactly do we remove them? How can we actively cleanse, rebuild, **and defend our bodies in a world filled with invisible threats?**

Enter the Clark Protocol—a practical, **accessible system for deep healing that integrates three core pillars:**

1. Herbal Cleanses to eliminate parasites and support detox organs.
2. The Zapper, a simple electrical device that disables pathogens.
3. Diet as a defensive strategy, where food becomes active medicine.

In this chapter, you'll learn how to integrate these elements into your life—and how this cookbook complements them every step of the way.

Herbal Cleanses: Liver, Kidney, and Parasite

Dr. Clark taught that parasites could only thrive in a body burdened by toxicity. Therefore, cleansing the body's filter organs—the liver and kidneys—is just as important as eliminating the parasites themselves.

She developed specific herbal protocols to do exactly that, starting with the parasite cleanse, followed by liver and kidney cleanses, each working synergistically with one another.

1. The Parasite Cleanse: Clearing the Invaders

The first and most critical step in the Clark Protocol is the parasite cleanse. **The goal is to eliminate all stages of the parasite lifecycle:** eggs, larvae, and adults.

Dr. Clark's three main antiparasitic herbs are:

- Black Walnut Hull (green) – Kills adult parasites.
- Wormwood (Artemisia absinthium) – Targets larval stages.
- Cloves (Syzygium aromaticum) – Destroys parasite eggs.

These herbs work best together, as they cover all stages of parasitic development.

Standard Clark Parasite Protocol (Simplified):

- **Black Walnut Tincture**: Begin with 1 drop in water and gradually increase the dose each day until reaching 2 teaspoons.
- **Wormwood Capsules**: Begin with 1 capsule/day, gradually increase to. 7.

- **Clove Capsules**: 3 capsules/day to kill parasite eggs.

Important: Be sure to consult your healthcare professional before beginning any herbal treatment.

This cleanse is typically run for 2–3 weeks, followed by maintenance doses. It can be repeated multiple times a year for ongoing protection.

2. Liver Cleanse: Unblocking the Body's Filter

The liver, responsible for filtering toxins and producing bile, often becomes congested with stones, fats, and parasite debris. A sluggish liver means toxins are recirculated and parasites gain a stronger foothold.

Dr. Clark's liver cleanse aims to flush gallstones and sludge, thereby restoring bile flow and digestive power.

Core Ingredients of the Clark Liver Flush:

- Fresh grapefruit or lemon juice
- Olive oil (extra virgin)
- Epsom salts (magnesium sulfate)
- Black walnut and parasite herbs (pre-flush prep)

Simplified Liver Flush Instructions:

1. Take parasite herbs for 5–7 days prior to the cleanse.
2. Fast after 2 PM on the day of the cleanse.
3. Take 1 tablespoon of Epsom salts mixed in water at 6 PM and again at 8 PM.
4. At 10 PM, drink a mix of ½ cup olive oil and ½ cup grapefruit juice.

5. Lie down immediately and stay still.
6. The following morning, consume two additional servings of Epsom salts.

Gallstones may be expelled the next day as small green or yellowish pellets in the stool.

Frequency: Once every 2–4 weeks during detox season or as needed.

3. Kidney Cleanse: Releasing the Backlog

The kidneys filter blood, regulate fluid balance, and eliminate acids and toxins. When overloaded, they struggle to perform. The Clark Kidney Cleanse uses gentle herbs and diuretics to dissolve kidney stones, reduce inflammation, and improve filtration.

Key Herbs for the Kidney Cleanse:

- Hydrangea root
- Gravel root
- Marshmallow root
- Goldenrod
- Ginger
- Uva Ursi
- Parsley (as tea or juice)

These herbs are typically brewed into a strong tea and taken daily for 2–3 weeks. Lemon water and magnesium support are also encouraged to prevent stone formation.

The Zapper: Theory and Construction

One of Dr. Clark's most controversial—but effective—tools is the Zapper, a small electronic device that uses low-voltage electrical pulses to disable parasites, bacteria, viruses, and fungi.

While this may sound unconventional, the idea is rooted in simple bioelectric principles.

The Theory Behind the Zapper

Every microorganism has a specific resonant frequency—just like a musical note. When exposed to a low current at this frequency, these organisms rupture or become inactive.

The Zapper produces a positive offset square wave that passes through body tissues, targeting and disabling pathogens while leaving human cells unharmed. Dr. Clark discovered that just 7 minutes of zapping, followed by two 20-minute intervals with 20-minute breaks in between, significantly reduced parasitic load in her patients.

How to Build a Basic Zapper

Materials Needed:

- 9V battery
- 555 timer chip
- Resistors, capacitors (per simple circuit design)
- Switch and LED
- Copper pipe handles (or wrist electrodes)

- Basic housing box

You can find open-source schematics online or purchase a pre-assembled unit. The device is easy to build for those with minimal electronics experience.

Usage:

- Hold copper handles (or apply wrist straps).
- Use the 7/20/20/20 method (7 minutes on, 20 off, repeat).
- Use daily during the cleansing process.

When to Use the Zapper

- During parasite cleanses
- During colds, infections, or fatigue
- After travel or exposure to contaminated food
- Regularly as a preventive measure

Caution: Do not use near a pacemaker or on young children without professional supervision.

Diet as Defense: Food as Medicine

The third leg of the Clark Protocol is the one this cookbook is built upon—using food strategically to fortify the body, prevent reinfection, and detoxify on a daily basis.

Dr. Clark believed food was the ultimate defense—and the most easily controlled factor in our environment. But only if it's clean, non-toxic, and biologically supportive.

Guiding Principles of a Clark-Friendly Diet

1. No Commercial Food Additives
    - Avoid MSG, aspartame, nitrates, BHT, and artificial dyes.
2. Organic, Unprocessed, Whole Foods
    - Vegetables, fruits, nuts, seeds, wild-caught fish, clean meats.
    - Avoid anything boxed, canned, or pre-seasoned.
3. Parasite-Fighting Foods
    - Garlic, clove, ginger, turmeric, black walnut, raw honey.
4. Liver-Supportive Foods
    - Beets, carrots, dandelion leaves, lemon-infused water, and olive oil.
5. Kidney-Cleansing Foods
    - Celery, parsley, watermelon, cucumber, and nettle infusion.
6. Anti-Fungal and Anti-Bacterial Foods
    - Coconut oil, oregano, thyme, onion, probiotic-rich foods.
7. Mold-Free Staples
    - Store grains and nuts in airtight containers.

- Avoid moldy bread, stale nuts, and aged cheese.
8. Distilled Water
    - Steer clear of both tap water and bottled water. Use distilled water for drinking and cooking.

Meal Timing and Preparation Tips

- Cook fresh daily, avoid leftovers stored too long.
- Use stainless steel, glass, or ceramic cookware.
- Never use aluminum foil or non-stick pans.
- Wash produce thoroughly, even if organic.
- Include cleansing teas and broths between meals.

Synergy: How These Elements Work Together

The true power of the Clark Protocol comes not from one element alone, but from their combined synergy.

- The herbs remove the parasites.
- The zapper disables remaining pathogens and disrupts reinfection.
- The cleanses open the body's detox pathways.
- The diet starves invaders and nourishes healing tissues.

When all systems are working in harmony, the body becomes inhospitable to disease and capable of regeneration.

What This Cookbook Will Help You Do

This cookbook was designed as a companion to the Clark Protocol. Every recipe, ingredient choice, **and preparation method honors Dr. Clark's principles:**

- Every meal aims to detox and heal.
- Every food is free of additives and contaminants.
- Every week is structured to support cleanse phases.

You'll find parasite-fighting breakfasts, kidney-cleansing teas, liver-flushing broths, and Zapper-friendly snacks that provide strength—not strain.

In Chapter 3, we'll walk you through "**Setting Up Your Healing Kitchen**"—removing the toxic tools, replacing common foods with safe alternatives, and creating a space that aligns with your body's healing journey.

But remember this core truth:

- "**Your body was designed to heal. Remove the invaders, clear the pathways, and feed it wisely—and healing will be the inevitable result."**
   — Inspired by Dr. Hulda Regehr Clark

Chapter 3: The Parasite-Free Pantry

Garlic & Clove Detox Broth

Ingredients (Serves 2):

- 4 cups distilled water
- 1 bulb garlic, peeled and crushed
- 1 tsp whole cloves
- 1 inch ginger root, sliced
- 1 tbsp olive oil
- ½ tsp Himalayan salt
- Juice of ½ lemon

Instructions:

1. Heat water in a saucepan until it reaches a boil.
2. Add garlic, cloves, and ginger. Simmer for 15–20 minutes.
3. Take off the heat, strain the mixture, then mix in olive oil, lemon juice, and salt.
4. Serve hot.

Nutritional Information (per serving):
Calories: 98
Protein: 1g
Fat: 8g
Carbohydrates: 6g
Fiber: 1.5g
Sugars: 0.5g
Sodium: 320mg

Black Walnut Green Smoothie

Ingredients (Serves 1):

- 1 cup kale leaves
- 1 green apple, chopped
- ½ banana
- ½ tsp black walnut tincture
- 1 tsp chia seeds
- 1 cup distilled water
- Ice (optional)

Instructions:

1. Add all ingredients to a blender.
2. Blend until smooth.
3. Serve immediately.

Nutritional Information (per serving):

Calories: 132

Protein: 2g

Fat: 4g

Carbohydrates: 25g

Fiber: 4g

Sugars: 13g

Sodium: 38mg

Spiced Pumpkin Seed Pesto

Ingredients (Serves 4):

- 1 cup raw pumpkin seeds
- 2 cups fresh basil leaves
- 3 cloves garlic
- ½ tsp ground clove
- ¼ cup olive oil
- 2 tbsp lemon juice
- ½ tsp salt

Instructions:

1. In a food processor, combine all ingredients.
2. Pulse until smooth.
3. Store in a glass jar. Use as spread or pasta topping.

Nutritional Information (per serving):

Calories: 210

Protein: 6g

Fat: 19g

Carbohydrates: 6g

Fiber: 2g

Sugars: 0g

Sodium: 200mg

Wormwood Tea Elixir

Ingredients (Serves 1):

- 1 cup distilled water
- ½ tsp dried wormwood leaves
- 1 tsp raw honey (optional)

Instructions:

1. Bring water to a boil.
2. Steep wormwood for 10 minutes.
3. Strain, add honey, and serve.

Nutritional Information (per serving):

Calories: 20 (without honey)

Protein: 0g

Fat: 0g

Carbohydrates: 5g

Fiber: 0g

Sugars: 5g (with honey)

Sodium: 0mg

Ginger-Cilantro Parasite Cleanse Soup

Ingredients (Serves 4):

- 4 cups vegetable broth (homemade, clean)
- 1 cup chopped celery
- 1 cup chopped carrots
- 2 cloves garlic, minced
- 2 inches ginger, grated
- ½ cup chopped cilantro
- 1 tbsp olive oil
- Salt to taste

Instructions:

1. In a large pot, warm the oil and sauté the garlic and ginger.
2. Add vegetables and broth. Simmer for 20 minutes.
3. Add cilantro and salt before serving.

Nutritional Information (per serving):

Calories: 90

Protein: 2g

Fat: 5g

Carbohydrates: 9g

Fiber: 2g

Sugars: 3g

Sodium: 300mg

Raw Garlic & Olive Tapenade

Ingredients (Serves 6):

- 1 cup green olives, pitted
- 4 cloves raw garlic
- 2 tbsp capers
- ¼ cup olive oil
- 2 tbsp lemon juice
- ¼ tsp ground clove

Instructions:

1. Blend all ingredients in a food processor.
2. Chill and serve as a spread or dip.

Nutritional Information (per serving):

Calories: 110

Protein: 1g

Fat: 10g

Carbohydrates: 3g

Fiber: 1g

Sugars: 0g

Sodium: 450mg

Clove-Infused Detox Rice

Ingredients (Serves 3):

- 1 cup organic basmati rice
- 2 cups distilled water
- ½ tsp ground cloves
- 1 tbsp coconut oil
- Pinch of salt

Instructions:

1. Rinse rice thoroughly.
2. In a saucepan, combine all ingredients.
3. Bring to a boil, then reduce heat and simmer for 15 minutes.
4. Let sit for 5 minutes before serving.

Nutritional Information (per serving):

Calories: 210

Protein: 3g

Fat: 5g

Carbohydrates: 38g

Fiber: 1g

Sugars: 0g

Sodium: 80mg

Turmeric-Parsley Detox Tonic

Ingredients (Serves 1):

- 1 cup distilled water
- ½ tsp turmeric powder
- 2 tbsp fresh parsley, chopped
- Juice of ½ lemon
- Pinch of cayenne

Instructions:

1. Mix all ingredients in warm water.
2. Let steep for 5 minutes. Drink warm or cool.

Nutritional Information (per serving):

Calories: 12

Protein: 0.5g

Fat: 0g

Carbohydrates: 2g

Fiber: 0.5g

Sugars: 0g

Sodium: 10mg

Raw Papaya Anti-Parasite Salad

Ingredients (Serves 2):

- 1 cup grated green papaya
- ½ cup cucumber, sliced
- 1 tbsp lime juice
- 1 tsp grated ginger
- 1 tsp olive oil
- Pinch of salt

Instructions:

1. Combine all ingredients in a bowl.
2. Toss and serve chilled.

Nutritional Information (per serving):

Calories: 45

Protein: 1g

Fat: 2g

Carbohydrates: 6g

Fiber: 2g

Sugars: 3g

Sodium: 50mg

Anti-Parasitic Spicy Carrot Juice

Ingredients (Serves 1):

- 3 large carrots
- 1 clove garlic
- 1 inch ginger
- ¼ tsp turmeric
- 1 cup water

Instructions:

1. Juice all ingredients or blend and strain.
2. Serve immediately.

Nutritional Information (per serving):

Calories: 90

Protein: 2g

Fat: 0.5g

Carbohydrates: 20g

Fiber: 3g

Sugars: 9g

Sodium: 70mg

Pumpkin Seed Snack Mix

Ingredients (Serves 4):

- 1 cup raw pumpkin seeds
- 1 tbsp coconut oil
- ¼ tsp sea salt
- ¼ tsp ground cloves
- ¼ tsp cayenne

Instructions:

1. Toss seeds in oil and spices.
2. Roast at 300°F for 20 minutes.
3. Cool and store in an airtight container.

Nutritional Information (per serving):

Calories: 160

Protein: 7g

Fat: 13g

Carbohydrates: 4g

Fiber: 2g

Sugars: 0g

Sodium: 150mg

Cabbage & Garlic Stir-Fry

Ingredients (Serves 3):

- 2 cups shredded green cabbage
- 3 cloves garlic, minced
- 1 tbsp olive oil
- ½ tsp cumin
- Salt to taste

Instructions:

1. Heat oil, sauté garlic for 1 minute.
2. Add cabbage and stir-fry 5–7 minutes.
3. Add cumin and salt before serving.

Nutritional Information (per serving):

Calories: 90

Protein: 2g

Fat: 7g

Carbohydrates: 6g

Fiber: 2g

Sugars: 2g

Sodium: 100mg

Anti-Parasitic Golden Milk

Ingredients (Serves 1):

- 1 cup coconut milk
- ½ tsp turmeric
- ¼ tsp ground clove
- 1 inch ginger
- 1 tsp raw honey (optional)

Instructions:

1. Warm coconut milk in a saucepan.
2. Add spices and simmer for 5 minutes.
3. Strain, stir in honey, and serve warm.

Nutritional Information (per serving):

Calories: 140

Protein: 1g

Fat: 12g

Carbohydrates: 6g

Fiber: 1g

Sugars: 4g

Sodium: 15mg

Zucchini & Clove Skillet

Ingredients (Serves 2):

- 2 small zucchinis, sliced
- 1 tbsp olive oil
- ¼ tsp ground cloves
- 2 garlic cloves, minced
- Salt to taste

Instructions:

1. Heat oil, sauté garlic for 1 minute.
2. Add zucchini and clove, cook until tender.
3. Salt to taste and serve.

Nutritional Information (per serving):

Calories: 85

Protein: 2g

Fat: 7g

Carbohydrates: 5g

Fiber: 2g

Sugars: 2g

Sodium: 60mg

Parasite-Cleansing Herb Omelet

Ingredients (Serves 1):

- 2 organic eggs
- 1 tbsp chopped parsley
- 1 tbsp chopped cilantro
- 1 clove garlic, minced
- 1 tbsp olive oil
- Salt to taste

Instructions:

1. Whisk eggs with herbs and garlic.
2. Warm the oil in a skillet, then add the mixture.
3. Cook 2–3 minutes per side. Serve hot.

Nutritional Information (per serving):

Calories: 215

Protein: 12g

Fat: 18g

Carbohydrates: 2g

Fiber: 0.5g

Sugars: 0g

Sodium: 200mg

Chapter 4: Liver and Kidney Loving Recipes

Beet & Carrot Liver Flush Juice

Ingredients (Serves 1):

- 1 medium beet, peeled and chopped
- 2 medium carrots
- 1 apple
- 1 inch ginger
- ½ lemon, juiced
- ½ cup distilled water

Instructions:

1. Juice the beet, carrots, apple, and ginger.
2. Stir in lemon juice and water.
3. Serve immediately.

Nutritional Information (per serving):

Calories: 135

Protein: 2g

Fat: 0g

Carbohydrates: 34g

Fiber: 5g

Sugars: 20g

Sodium: 100mg

Dandelion Greens & Apple Salad

Ingredients (Serves 2):

- 2 cups dandelion greens, chopped
- 1 green apple, thinly sliced
- 1 tbsp lemon juice
- 1 tbsp olive oil
- ½ tsp raw honey
- Pinch of sea salt

Instructions:

1. In a bowl, mix lemon juice, olive oil, honey, and salt.
2. Toss dandelion greens and apples in dressing.
3. Serve fresh.

Nutritional Information (per serving):

Calories: 95

Protein: 1g

Fat: 7g

Carbohydrates: 10g

Fiber: 3g

Sugars: 6g

Sodium: 45mg

Parsley-Lemon Detox Tea

Ingredients (Serves 1):

- 1 cup boiling distilled water
- 1 tbsp chopped fresh parsley
- Juice of ½ lemon
- Optional: pinch of cayenne

Instructions:

1. Let the parsley steep in hot boiling water for 10 minutes.
2. Strain and stir in lemon juice.
3. Add cayenne if desired. Drink warm.

Nutritional Information (per serving):

Calories: 5

Protein: 0g

Fat: 0g

Carbohydrates: 1g

Fiber: 0g

Sugars: 0g

Sodium: 5mg

Turmeric & Ginger Kidney Broth

Ingredients (Serves 2):

- 4 cups distilled water
- 1 inch fresh turmeric root, sliced
- 1 inch fresh ginger root, sliced
- 2 garlic cloves, crushed
- ½ tsp sea salt

Instructions:

1. In a pot, combine all ingredients.
2. Simmer on low heat for 25 minutes.
3. Strain and serve warm.

Nutritional Information (per serving):

Calories: 20

Protein: 0g

Fat: 0g

Carbohydrates: 4g

Fiber: 0.5g

Sugars: 0g

Sodium: 260mg

Watermelon-Cucumber Kidney Flush

Ingredients (Serves 1):

- 1 cup diced watermelon
- ½ cucumber, sliced
- Juice of ½ lime
- 4 fresh mint leaves
- ½ cup distilled water

Instructions:

1. Blend all ingredients until smooth.
2. Strain if desired and serve cold.

Nutritional Information (per serving):

Calories: 45

Protein: 1g

Fat: 0g

Carbohydrates: 11g

Fiber: 1g

Sugars: 9g

Sodium: 5mg

Celery & Apple Juice for Kidneys

Ingredients (Serves 1):

- 2 celery stalks
- 1 green apple
- ½ lemon, juiced
- ½ cup cold distilled water

Instructions:

1. Juice celery and apple.
2. Stir in lemon juice and water.
3. Serve fresh.

Nutritional Information (per serving):

Calories: 60

Protein: 1g

Fat: 0g

Carbohydrates: 14g

Fiber: 2g

Sugars: 10g

Sodium: 75mg

Cilantro-Pumpkin Seed Liver Salad

Ingredients (Serves 2):

- 2 cups mixed greens
- ¼ cup chopped cilantro
- 2 tbsp raw pumpkin seeds
- 1 tbsp olive oil
- 1 tbsp apple cider vinegar
- Pinch of pink salt

Instructions:

1. Mix greens and cilantro in a bowl.
2. Top with seeds.
3. Whisk oil, vinegar, and salt; drizzle over salad.

Nutritional Information (per serving):

Calories: 140

Protein: 4g

Fat: 12g

Carbohydrates: 4g

Fiber: 2g

Sugars: 0g

Sodium: 90mg

Kidney Tea Blend

Ingredients (Serves 1):

- 1 tsp dried nettle leaves
- 1 tsp dried hydrangea root
- 1 tsp dried marshmallow root
- 1½ cups boiling distilled water

Instructions:

1. Place the herbs into a tea strainer or teabag.
2. Steep in boiling water for 15 minutes.
3. Remove herbs and drink warm.

Nutritional Information (per serving):

Calories: 8

Protein: 0g

Fat: 0g

Carbohydrates: 2g

Fiber: 0g

Sugars: 0g

Sodium: 0mg

Bitter Greens Liver Bowl

Ingredients (Serves 2):

- 1 cup chopped arugula
- 1 cup chopped endive
- ½ avocado, sliced
- 1 tbsp lemon juice
- 1 tbsp cold-pressed flax oil
- 1 tbsp hemp seeds

Instructions:

1. Combine greens in a bowl.
2. Add avocado and hemp seeds.
3. Drizzle with lemon juice and oil.

Nutritional Information (per serving):

Calories: 180

Protein: 3g

Fat: 15g

Carbohydrates: 6g

Fiber: 4g

Sugars: 0g

Sodium: 40mg

Golden Kidney & Liver Soup

Ingredients (Serves 4):

- 4 cups vegetable broth
- 1 cup chopped zucchini
- 1 cup chopped carrots
- 1 onion, diced
- 1 tsp turmeric powder
- 1 tsp ground cumin
- 2 tbsp olive oil

Instructions:

1. In a pot, heat oil and sauté onion.
2. Add all vegetables, spices, and broth.
3. Simmer for 20–25 minutes. Serve warm.

Nutritional Information (per serving):

Calories: 110

Protein: 2g

Fat: 7g

Carbohydrates: 10g

Fiber: 2g

Sugars: 4g

Sodium: 280mg

Cucumber-Mint Detox Water

Ingredients (Serves 2):

- 4 cups distilled water
- ½ cucumber, thinly sliced
- 5 fresh mint leaves
- Juice of ½ lemon

Instructions:

1. Combine all ingredients in a glass pitcher.
2. Chill for 1 hour before serving.

Nutritional Information (per serving):

Calories: 2

Protein: 0g

Fat: 0g

Carbohydrates: 0.5g

Fiber: 0g

Sugars: 0g

Sodium: 1mg

Milk Thistle Smoothie

Ingredients (Serves 1):

- 1 cup unsweetened almond milk
- 1 tbsp ground milk thistle seeds
- ½ banana
- ½ cup blueberries
- 1 tbsp chia seeds

Instructions:

1. Blend all ingredients until smooth.
2. Serve immediately.

Nutritional Information (per serving):

Calories: 165

Protein: 4g

Fat: 9g

Carbohydrates: 20g

Fiber: 6g

Sugars: 9g

Sodium: 90mg

Liver-Loving Sweet Potato Mash

Ingredients (Serves 2):

- 1 large sweet potato, peeled and cubed
- 1 tbsp coconut oil
- 1 tsp turmeric powder
- Salt to taste

Instructions:

1. Boil sweet potato until soft.
2. Mash with coconut oil, turmeric, and salt.
3. Serve warm.

Nutritional Information (per serving):

Calories: 150

Protein: 2g

Fat: 7g

Carbohydrates: 22g

Fiber: 3g

Sugars: 6g

Sodium: 70mg

Herbal Kidney Detox Infusion

Ingredients (Serves 1):

- 1 tsp uva ursi leaves
- 1 tsp dried goldenrod
- 1½ cups boiling distilled water

Instructions:

1. Infuse the herbs in boiling water for 10 to 15 minutes.
2. Strain and drink 1 cup daily.

Nutritional Facts (per serving):

Calories: 5

Protein: 0g

Total Fat: 0g

Carbohydrates: 1g

Dietary Fiber: 0g

Sugars: 0g

Sodium: 0mg

Lemon-Olive Oil Liver Shot

Ingredients (Serves 1):

- 1 tbsp extra virgin olive oil
- Juice of ½ lemon
- Pinch of cayenne pepper

Instructions:

1. Whisk all ingredients in a small cup.
2. Drink first thing in the morning on an empty stomach.

Nutritional Information (per serving):

Calories: 120

Protein: 0g

Fat: 14g

Carbohydrates: 1g

Fiber: 0g

Sugars: 0g

Sodium: 1mg

Chapter 5: Heavy Metal Detox Dishes

Cilantro-Lime Quinoa Bowl

Ingredients (Serves 2):

- 1 cup cooked quinoa
- ½ cup chopped fresh cilantro
- 1 avocado, diced
- 1 tbsp olive oil
- Juice of 1 lime
- ½ tsp sea salt

Instructions:

1. Cook quinoa according to the package. Let cool.
2. Mix cilantro, avocado, lime juice, olive oil, and salt into quinoa.
3. Serve chilled or at room temperature.

Nutritional Information (per serving):

Calories: 310

Protein: 7g

Fat: 18g

Carbohydrates: 28g

Fiber: 6g

Sugars: 1g

Sodium: 290mg

Chlorella Green Detox Smoothie

Ingredients (Serves 1):

- 1 cup spinach
- ½ banana
- ½ green apple
- 1 tsp chlorella powder
- 1 tbsp flaxseed
- 1 cup unsweetened almond milk

Instructions:

1. Blend all ingredients until smooth.
2. Drink immediately.

Nutritional Information (per serving):

Calories: 160

Protein: 3g

Fat: 5g

Carbohydrates: 23g

Fiber: 5g

Sugars: 10g

Sodium: 90mg

Garlic & Broccoli Stir-Fry

Ingredients (Serves 2):

- 2 cups broccoli florets
- 3 garlic cloves, minced
- 1 tbsp coconut oil
- 1 tbsp tamari (gluten-free soy sauce)
- ½ tsp ground ginger

Instructions:

1. Heat oil in a skillet. Add garlic and ginger.
2. Add broccoli and stir-fry for 5–7 minutes.
3. Add tamari, stir, and serve.

Nutritional Information (per serving):

Calories: 110

Protein: 4g

Fat: 7g

Carbohydrates: 9g

Fiber: 3g

Sugars: 2g

Sodium: 320mg

Cilantro-Pumpkin Seed Pesto Pasta

Ingredients (Serves 2):

- 1½ cups cooked gluten-free pasta
- 1 cup cilantro
- 2 tbsp pumpkin seeds
- 1 tbsp olive oil
- 1 garlic clove
- Juice of ½ lemon

Instructions:

1. Blend together cilantro, seeds, oil, garlic, and lemon to create a pesto.
2. Toss pesto with warm pasta.
3. Serve immediately.

Nutritional Information (per serving):

Calories: 300

Protein: 7g

Fat: 13g

Carbohydrates: 35g

Fiber: 4g

Sugars: 1g

Sodium: 90mg

Seaweed & Avocado Wraps

Ingredients (Serves 1):

- 2 nori sheets
- ½ avocado, sliced
- ¼ cup shredded carrots
- ¼ cup alfalfa sprouts
- 1 tbsp tahini
- 1 tsp lemon juice

Instructions:

1. Spread tahini and lemon on nori sheets.
2. Add avocado, carrots, and sprouts.
3. Roll tightly and slice.

Nutritional Information (per serving):

Calories: 190

Protein: 4g

Fat: 13g

Carbohydrates: 14g

Fiber: 6g

Sugars: 1g

Sodium: 150mg

Brazil Nut & Spinach Salad

Ingredients (Serves 2):

- 2 cups spinach
- 4 Brazil nuts, chopped
- ½ cup cucumber slices
- 2 tbsp olive oil
- Juice of ½ orange
- Sea salt to taste

Instructions:

1. Mix spinach, cucumber, and Brazil nuts.
2. Drizzle with oil and orange juice.
3. Toss and serve.

Nutritional Information (per serving):

Calories: 210

Protein: 3g

Fat: 20g

Carbohydrates: 6g

Fiber: 2g

Sugars: 2g

Sodium: 50mg

Selenium: 100+ mcg

Cilantro Detox Dressing

Ingredients (Serves 2):

- 1 cup fresh cilantro
- ¼ cup olive oil
- 1 garlic clove
- Juice of 1 lemon
- ½ tsp sea salt

Instructions:

1. Blend all ingredients until creamy.
2. Use on salads or cooked veggies.

Nutritional Information (per serving):

Calories: 120

Protein: 0g

Fat: 14g

Carbohydrates: 1g

Fiber: 0g

Sugars: 0g

Sodium: 240mg

Sweet Potato & Parsley Mash

Ingredients (Serves 2):

- 1 large sweet potato
- 2 tbsp chopped parsley
- 1 tbsp coconut oil
- ¼ tsp sea salt

Instructions:

1. Boil sweet potato until tender.
2. Mash with coconut oil, parsley, and salt.
3. Serve warm.

Nutritional Information (per serving):

Calories: 160

Protein: 2g

Fat: 7g

Carbohydrates: 24g

Fiber: 3g

Sugars: 5g

Sodium: 150mg

Spirulina Detox Shot

Ingredients (Serves 1):

- ½ tsp spirulina powder
- ½ cup cold distilled water
- Juice of ½ lemon

Instructions:

1. Mix all ingredients in a small glass.
2. Drink immediately on an empty stomach.

Nutritional Information (per serving):

Calories: 20

Protein: 2g

Fat: 0g

Carbohydrates: 1g

Fiber: 0g

Sugars: 0g

Sodium: 10mg

Bok Choy & Garlic Stir Fry

Ingredients (Serves 2):

- 3 cups chopped bok choy
- 2 garlic cloves, minced
- 1 tbsp avocado oil
- 1 tbsp tamari

Instructions:

1. Heat oil in a pan and sauté garlic.
2. Add bok choy and tamari. Cook for 5 minutes.
3. Serve hot.

Nutritional Information (per serving):

Calories: 90

Protein: 3g

Fat: 6g

Carbohydrates: 7g

Fiber: 2g

Sugars: 2g

Sodium: 280mg

Detox Lentil & Cilantro Soup

Ingredients (Serves 3):

- 1 cup cooked lentils
- 2 cups veggie broth
- ½ cup chopped cilantro
- 1 garlic clove, minced
- ½ onion, diced

Instructions:

1. Sauté onion and garlic in 1 tsp olive oil.
2. Add lentils, broth, and cilantro.
3. Simmer for 15 minutes and serve.

Nutritional Information (per serving):

Calories: 160

Protein: 9g

Fat: 3g

Carbohydrates: 23g

Fiber: 7g

Sugars: 2g

Sodium: 320mg

Lemon-Ginger Detox Water

Ingredients (Serves 2):

- 4 cups distilled water
- 1 inch fresh ginger, sliced
- Juice of 1 lemon

Instructions:

1. Combine ingredients and let infuse for 30 minutes.
2. Drink throughout the day.

Nutrition Facts (per serving):

Calories: 4

Protein: 0g

Fat: 0g

Carbohydrates: 1g

Fiber: 0g

Sugar: 0g

Sodium: 0mg

Chlorella Energy Balls

Ingredients (Makes 6 Balls, Serves 3):

- ½ cup sunflower seeds
- ½ cup pitted dates
- 1 tsp chlorella powder
- 1 tbsp almond butter
- 1 tbsp shredded coconut

Instructions:

1. Pulse all ingredients in a food processor.
2. Roll into small balls and refrigerate.
3. Eat 2 per serving.

Nutritional Information (per serving of 2 balls):

Calories: 180

Protein: 4g

Fat: 9g

Carbohydrates: 22g

Fiber: 3g

Sugars: 16g

Sodium: 5mg

Heavy Metal Detox Soup

Ingredients (Serves 3):

- 1 cup chopped celery
- 1 cup zucchini
- 1 cup cauliflower
- 1 garlic clove
- 1 tsp turmeric
- 3 cups vegetable broth
- ½ cup chopped parsley

Instructions:

1. Simmer all ingredients in broth for 20 minutes.
2. Blend for a creamy texture if desired.
3. Serve hot.

Nutritional Information (per serving):

Calories: 85

Protein: 3g

Fat: 2g

Carbohydrates: 14g

Fiber: 4g

Sugars: 3g

Sodium: 300mg

Cilantro & Green Apple Juice

Ingredients (Serves 1):

- 1 cup cilantro
- 1 green apple
- ½ cucumber
- Juice of ½ lemon
- ½ cup water

Instructions:

1. Juice all ingredients or blend and strain.
2. Serve chilled.

Nutritional Information (per serving):

Calories: 65

Protein: 1g

Fat: 0g

Carbohydrates: 16g

Fiber: 3g

Sugars: 12g

Sodium: 20mg

Chapter 6: Immune-Strengthening Meals

Immunity Boosting Garlic & Turmeric Soup

Ingredients (Serves 2):

- 1 tbsp olive oil
- 4 garlic cloves, minced
- 1 small onion, chopped
- 1 tsp ground turmeric
- 2 cups vegetable broth
- ½ cup coconut milk
- Sea salt and pepper to taste

Instructions:

1. Sauté garlic and onion in olive oil for 3 minutes.
2. Add turmeric and cook for 1 minute.
3. Pour in broth and coconut milk.
4. Simmer for 10 minutes.
5. Blend if desired for creamy texture.

Per Serving Nutritional Values:

Calories: 165

Protein: 2g

Fat: 13g

Carbohydrates: 10g

Fiber: 2g

Sugar: 2g

Sodium: 340mg

Ginger-Miso Immunity Broth

Ingredients (Serves 2):

- 2 cups water
- 1 tbsp miso paste
- 1-inch ginger, grated
- 1 garlic clove, minced
- 1 tbsp chopped scallions
- ¼ cup chopped shiitake mushrooms

Instructions:

1. Simmer the water with ginger, garlic, and mushrooms for 10 minutes.
2. Turn off heat, stir in miso paste.
3. Top with scallions and serve.

Nutritional Information (per serving):

Calories: 60

Protein: 2g

Fat: 1g

Carbohydrates: 9g

Fiber: 1g

Sugars: 1g

Sodium: 620mg

Vitamin C Super Smoothie

Ingredients (Serves 1):

- 1 orange, peeled
- ½ cup strawberries
- ½ kiwi
- 1 tbsp chia seeds
- ½ cup water or coconut water

Instructions:

1. Blend all ingredients until smooth.
2. Drink immediately for best results.

Nutritional Information (per serving):

Calories: 130

Protein: 2g

Fat: 4g

Carbohydrates: 24g

Fiber: 6g

Sugars: 14g

Sodium: 5mg

Vitamin C: 120% DV

Immune Greens Stir-Fry

Ingredients (Serves 2):

- 2 cups kale, chopped
- 1 cup broccoli florets
- 1 garlic clove, minced
- 1 tbsp sesame oil
- 1 tbsp tamari

Instructions:

1. Heat sesame oil in a pan, add garlic.
2. Stir-fry kale and broccoli for 5 minutes.
3. Add tamari and cook for 2 more minutes.

Nutritional Information (per serving):

Calories: 110

Protein: 4g

Fat: 7g

Carbohydrates: 8g

Fiber: 3g

Sugars: 1g

Sodium: 370mg

Zinc-Packed Pumpkin Seed Porridge

Ingredients (Serves 1):

- ½ cup cooked oats
- 1 tbsp ground pumpkin seeds
- 1 tbsp flaxseed
- 1 tsp cinnamon
- 1 tsp raw honey
- ½ cup unsweetened almond milk

Instructions:

1. Mix all ingredients in a bowl.
2. Warm slightly if desired or serve cold.

Nutritional Information (per serving):

Calories: 220

Protein: 6g

Fat: 9g

Carbohydrates: 28g

Fiber: 5g

Sugars: 6g

Sodium: 45mg

Zinc: 12% DV

Citrus-Garlic Immunity Shot

Ingredients (Serves 1):

- Juice of 1 lemon
- 1 garlic clove, crushed
- ½ tsp turmeric powder
- ⅛ tsp cayenne
- 1 tsp raw honey

Instructions:

1. Mix all ingredients well.
2. Drink quickly like a shot.

Nutritional Information (per serving):

Calories: 35

Protein: 0g

Fat: 0g

Carbohydrates: 9g

Fiber: 0g

Sugars: 7g

Vitamin C: 90% DV

Fermented Veggie Bowl

Ingredients (Serves 1):

- ½ cup cooked brown rice
- ¼ cup sauerkraut (unpasteurized)
- ½ avocado, sliced
- 1 tbsp pumpkin seeds
- 1 tbsp olive oil

Instructions:

1. Arrange rice in a bowl.
2. Add sauerkraut, avocado, and seeds.
3. Drizzle with olive oil.

Nutritional Information (per serving):

Calories: 280

Protein: 5g

Fat: 18g

Carbohydrates: 22g

Fiber: 5g

Sugars: 1g

Sodium: 300mg

Probiotics: Yes

Reishi Mushroom Tea

Ingredients (Serves 1):

- 1 cup hot water
- 1 tsp dried reishi mushroom powder
- ½ tsp cinnamon
- Optional: 1 tsp raw honey

Instructions:

1. Steep all ingredients in hot water for 10 minutes.
2. Strain and sip slowly.

Nutritional Information (per serving):

Calories: 20

Protein: 0g

Fat: 0g

Carbohydrates: 5g

Fiber: 0g

Sugars: 4g (if honey added)

Immunity Garden Salad

Ingredients (Serves 2):

- 2 cups mixed greens
- ½ cup shredded carrots
- ½ cup purple cabbage
- ¼ cup red bell pepper
- 1 tbsp sunflower seeds
- 1 tbsp apple cider vinegar
- 1 tbsp olive oil

Instructions:

1. Combine all vegetables and seeds in a bowl and toss to mix.
2. Drizzle with vinegar and olive oil.
3. Serve fresh.

Nutrition Information (per serving):

Calories: 140

Protein: 3g

Fat: 10g

Carbohydrates: 10g

Fiber: 3g

Sugar: 5g

Sodium: 50mg

Garlic-Lemon Roasted Cauliflower

Ingredients (Serves 2):

- 2 cups cauliflower florets
- 1 tbsp olive oil
- 2 garlic cloves, minced
- Juice of ½ lemon
- Sea salt to taste

Instructions:

1. Preheat the oven to 400°F (200°C).
2. Toss cauliflower with oil, garlic, lemon, and salt.
3. Roast 25 minutes, turning once.

Nutritional Information (per serving):

Calories: 120

Protein: 3g

Fat: 8g

Carbohydrates: 10g

Fiber: 4g

Sugars: 2g

Sodium: 120mg

Turmeric Lentil Stew

Ingredients (Serves 2):

- ½ cup dry lentils
- 2 cups vegetable broth
- 1 carrot, diced
- 1 tsp turmeric
- 1 garlic clove, minced
- 1 tbsp olive oil

Instructions:

1. Sauté garlic in olive oil.
2. Add lentils, broth, carrot, and turmeric.
3. Simmer for 25–30 minutes until soft.

Nutritional Information (per serving):

Calories: 210

Protein: 11g

Fat: 7g

Carbohydrates: 27g

Fiber: 6g

Sugars: 3g

Sodium: 350mg

Green Immunity Juice

Ingredients (Serves 1):

- 1 cup spinach
- ½ green apple
- ½ cucumber
- Juice of ½ lemon
- 1 inch ginger root
- ½ cup water

Instructions:

1. Juice all ingredients or blend and strain.
2. Drink fresh.

Nutritional Information (per serving):

Calories: 60

Protein: 1g

Fat: 0g

Carbohydrates: 15g

Fiber: 3g

Sugars: 10g

Sodium: 15mg

Sesame-Garlic Bok Choy

Ingredients (Serves 2):

- 2 cups bok choy, chopped
- 1 tbsp sesame oil
- 2 garlic cloves, minced
- 1 tbsp tamari

Instructions:

1. Warm the oil in a skillet and sauté the garlic.
2. Add bok choy and cook for 5 minutes.
3. Add tamari and cook for 2 more minutes.

Nutritional Information (per serving):

Calories: 100

Protein: 2g

Fat: 8g

Carbohydrates: 6g

Fiber: 2g

Sugars: 2g

Sodium: 320mg

Yogurt-Parfait Power Cup

Ingredients (Serves 1):

- ½ cup plain unsweetened coconut yogurt (or probiotic-rich yogurt)
- ¼ cup blueberries
- 1 tbsp ground flaxseed
- 1 tsp raw honey

Instructions:

1. Layer yogurt with berries and flaxseed.
2. Drizzle with honey.
3. Chill and serve.

Nutritional Details (per serving):

Calories: 140

Protein: 2g

Fat: 6g

Carbohydrates: 19g

Fiber: 4g

Sugar: 12g

Contains Probiotics: Yes

Spiced Golden Milk Latte

Ingredients (Serves 1):

- 1 cup unsweetened almond milk
- ½ tsp turmeric
- ¼ tsp cinnamon
- Pinch of black pepper
- 1 tsp coconut oil
- 1 tsp raw honey

Instructions:

1. Heat all ingredients in a saucepan (do not boil).
2. Whisk well and pour into a mug.
3. Sip warm.

Nutritional Information (per serving):

Calories: 130

Protein: 1g

Fat: 10g

Carbohydrates: 10g

Fiber: 1g

Sugars: 6g

Sodium: 150mg

Chapter 7: Alkalizing and Anti-Mold Recipes

Alkaline Green Juice

Ingredients (Serves 1):

- 1 cup cucumber, chopped
- 1 celery stalk
- ½ green apple
- 1 handful parsley
- ½ lemon (juice only)
- ½ cup water

Instructions:

1. Blend all ingredients until smooth.
2. Strain or drink as-is.
3. Consume immediately.

Nutritional Information (per serving):

Calories: 40

Protein: 1g

Fat: 0g

Carbohydrates: 10g

Fiber: 2g

Sugars: 6g

Sodium: 25mg

pH effect: Alkalizing

Avocado-Cucumber Soup (Raw & Chilled)

Ingredients (Serves 2):

- 1 avocado
- 1 cup cucumber, peeled and diced
- ½ cup coconut water
- 1 tbsp lemon juice
- 1 garlic clove
- Pinch of Himalayan salt

Instructions:

1. Blend all ingredients until creamy.
2. Chill for 15 minutes.
3. Serve cold in bowls.

Nutritional Information (per serving):

Calories: 160

Protein: 2g

Fat: 14g

Carbohydrates: 8g

Fiber: 5g

Sugars: 2g

Sodium: 80mg

pH effect: Strongly Alkalizing

Quinoa Detox Bowl

Ingredients (Serves 2):

- 1 cup cooked quinoa
- ½ cup steamed kale
- ¼ cup grated beet
- ¼ avocado, sliced
- 1 tbsp lemon juice
- 1 tbsp olive oil

Instructions:

1. In a bowl, layer quinoa, kale, beet, and avocado.
2. Drizzle with lemon juice and olive oil.
3. Serve warm or cold.

Nutritional Information (per serving):

Calories: 220

Protein: 6g

Fat: 10g

Carbohydrates: 25g

Fiber: 6g

Sugars: 3g

Sodium: 45mg

pH effect: Alkalizing

Steamed Broccoli with Garlic-Oregano Oil

Ingredients (Serves 2):

- 2 cups broccoli florets
- 1 tbsp olive oil
- 1 garlic clove, minced
- ¼ tsp dried oregano

Instructions:

1. Steam broccoli until tender (5–6 min).
2. In a pan, heat oil and sauté garlic and oregano.
3. Drizzle over steamed broccoli and serve.

Nutritional Information (per serving):

Calories: 100

Protein: 4g

Fat: 7g

Carbohydrates: 8g

Fiber: 4g

Sugars: 2g

Sodium: 30mg

pH effect: Strongly Alkalizing

Zucchini Noodles with Basil-Pumpkin Seed Pesto

Ingredients (Serves 2):

- 2 medium zucchinis, spiralized
- ¼ cup pumpkin seeds
- 1 cup fresh basil
- 2 tbsp olive oil
- 1 garlic clove
- Juice of ½ lemon

Instructions:

1. Blend seeds, basil, oil, garlic, and lemon into pesto.
2. Toss zucchini noodles with pesto.
3. Serve raw or lightly warmed.

Nutritional Information (per serving):

Calories: 210

Protein: 5g

Fat: 17g

Carbohydrates: 10g

Fiber: 4g

Sugars: 3g

Sodium: 15mg

pH effect: Alkalizing & Antifungal

Anti-Mold Cabbage Slaw

Ingredients (Serves 2):

- 1 cup shredded green cabbage
- 1 cup shredded purple cabbage
- 1 tbsp lemon juice
- 1 tbsp apple cider vinegar
- 1 tbsp olive oil
- ½ tsp ground caraway seeds

Instructions:

1. Combine all ingredients in a large bowl.
2. Mix thoroughly and allow it to rest for 10 minutes.
3. Serve chilled.

Nutritional Information (per serving):

Calories: 90

Protein: 1g

Fat: 7g

Carbohydrates: 7g

Fiber: 3g

Sugars: 3g

Sodium: 40mg

pH effect: Alkalizing

Lemon-Thyme Roasted Carrots

Ingredients (Serves 2):

- 2 cups carrots, sliced
- 1 tbsp olive oil
- Juice of ½ lemon
- ½ tsp dried thyme

Instructions:

1. Preheat the oven to 375°F (190°C).
2. Toss carrots with oil, lemon, and thyme.
3. Roast for 30 minutes until tender.

Nutritional Information (per serving):

Calories: 110

Protein: 1g

Fat: 7g

Carbohydrates: 11g

Fiber: 3g

Sugars: 5g

Sodium: 50mg

pH effect: Alkalizing

Alkaline Seed Crackers

Ingredients (Serves 4):

- ¼ cup chia seeds
- ¼ cup flaxseeds
- ¼ cup sunflower seeds
- ¼ tsp Himalayan salt
- ½ cup water

Instructions:

1. Mix all ingredients and let sit for 15 minutes.
2. Spread onto parchment and dehydrate at 150°F for 4–6 hours.
3. Break into crackers and store dry.

Nutritional Information (per serving):

Calories: 150

Protein: 5g

Fat: 10g

Carbohydrates: 10g

Fiber: 6g

Sugars: 1g

Sodium: 90mg

pH effect: Alkalizing & Mold-Free

Fennel & Arugula Detox Salad

Ingredients (Serves 2):

- 1 cup arugula
- 1 cup shaved fennel
- 1 tbsp lemon juice
- 1 tbsp olive oil
- Pinch of salt

Instructions:

1. Toss fennel and arugula together.
2. Drizzle with lemon and oil.
3. Mix and serve immediately.

Nutritional Information (per serving):

Calories: 85

Protein: 1g

Fat: 7g

Carbohydrates: 5g

Fiber: 2g

Sugars: 2g

Sodium: 35mg

pH effect: Alkalizing

Turmeric-Almond Milk Tonic

Ingredients (Serves 1):

- 1 cup unsweetened almond milk
- ½ tsp turmeric
- Pinch of black pepper
- ½ tsp cinnamon
- 1 tsp raw honey (optional)

Instructions:

1. Warm almond milk and whisk in spices.
2. Stir in honey (optional).
3. Drink warm.

Nutritional Information (per serving):

Calories: 90

Protein: 1g

Fat: 6g

Carbohydrates: 9g

Fiber: 1g

Sugars: 6g

Sodium: 120mg

pH effect: Mildly Alkalizing

Mold-Free Coconut Yogurt Parfait

Ingredients (Serves 1):

- ½ cup plain coconut yogurt
- ¼ cup fresh blueberries
- 1 tbsp hemp seeds

Instructions:

1. Layer yogurt, berries, and seeds.
2. Serve chilled.

Nutritional Information (per serving):

Calories: 180

Protein: 3g

Fat: 12g

Carbohydrates: 12g

Fiber: 3g

Sugars: 5g

Sodium: 20mg

pH effect: Alkalizing & Probiotic

Cucumber-Mint Detox Water

Ingredients (Serves 2):

- 1 quart filtered water
- 6 cucumber slices
- 6 mint leaves
- 2 lemon slices

Instructions:

1. Add all ingredients to water.
2. Chill for 2 hours before serving.

Nutritional Information (per serving):

Calories: 5

Protein: 0g

Fat: 0g

Carbohydrates: 1g

Fiber: 0g

Sugars: 0g

Sodium: 2mg

pH effect: Strongly Alkalizing

Ginger-Lime Marinated Mushrooms

Ingredients (Serves 2):

- 1 cup button mushrooms, sliced
- 1 tbsp olive oil
- 1 tbsp lime juice
- ½ tsp grated ginger
- 1 garlic clove, minced

Instructions:

1. Mix all marinade ingredients.
2. Toss with mushrooms and marinate 1 hour.
3. Serve chilled or at room temperature.

Nutritional Information (per serving):

Calories: 95

Protein: 2g

Fat: 8g

Carbohydrates: 4g

Fiber: 1g

Sugars: 1g

Sodium: 20mg

pH effect: Alkalizing & Antifungal

Baked Lemon-Cilantro Cauliflower Rice

Ingredients (Serves 2):

- 2 cups cauliflower rice
- 1 tbsp olive oil
- Juice of ½ lemon
- 1 tbsp chopped cilantro

Instructions:

1. Toss all ingredients in a bowl.
2. Bake at 375°F (190°C) for 20 minutes.
3. Serve hot or cold.

Nutritional Information (per serving):

Calories: 95

Protein: 3g

Fat: 7g

Carbohydrates: 6g

Fiber: 3g

Sugars: 2g

Sodium: 40mg

pH effect: Alkalizing

Mold-Free Alkaline Veggie Stir-Fry

Ingredients (Serves 2):

- 1 cup chopped zucchini
- ½ cup snow peas
- ½ cup red bell pepper
- 1 tbsp coconut oil
- 1 tsp grated ginger
- 1 tbsp coconut aminos

Instructions:

1. Heat coconut oil and sauté ginger.
2. Add all vegetables and stir-fry 5–6 min.
3. Add coconut aminos and serve warm.

Nutritional Information (per serving):

Calories: 130

Protein: 2g

Fat: 10g

Carbohydrates: 8g

Fiber: 3g

Sugars: 3g

Sodium: 160mg

pH effect: Alkalizing & Mold-Free

Bonus Chapter : 30 Day Meal Plan

Week 1

DAY 1

Breakfast: Coconut Yogurt Parfait (Free from mold)

Lunch: Detox Quinoa Bowl

Dinner: Alkaline Vegetable Stir-Fry (Mold-free)

Snack: Mint and Cucumber Detox Water

DAY 2

Breakfast: Turmeric-Almond Milk Tonic

Lunch: Fennel & Arugula Detox Salad

Dinner: Garlic-Ginger Steamed Salmon (Immune recipe)

Snack: Alkaline Seed Crackers

DAY 3

Breakfast: Alkaline Green Juice

Lunch: Zucchini Noodles with Basil-Pumpkin Seed Pesto

Dinner: Baked Lemon-Cilantro Cauliflower Rice + Steamed Broccoli with Garlic-Oregano Oil

Snack: Ginger-Lime Marinated Mushrooms

🗒 DAY 4

Breakfast: Detox Apple Chia Bowl (Parasite-Free recipe)

Lunch: Warm Kale & Quinoa Detox Salad (Liver recipe)

Dinner: Roasted Beet & Garlic Soup (Liver recipe)

Snack: Cucumber-Mint Detox Water

🗒 DAY 5

Breakfast: Mold-Free Coconut Yogurt Parfait

Lunch: Turmeric-Cauliflower Rice Bowl (Heavy Metal Detox)

Dinner: Lemon-Thyme Roasted Carrots + Baked Wild Cod with Parsley (Kidney recipe)

Snack: Alkaline Seed Crackers

🗒 DAY 6

Breakfast: Turmeric-Almond Milk Tonic

Lunch: Lentil and Kale Stew (Heavy Metal Detox)

Dinner: Mold-Free Alkaline Veggie Stir-Fry

Snack: Fennel & Arugula Detox Salad

🗒 DAY 7

Breakfast: Alkaline Green Juice

Lunch: Cabbage Detox Soup (Liver recipe)

Dinner: Spaghetti Squash with Garlic-Basil Sauce (Immune recipe)

Snack: Ginger-Lime Marinated Mushrooms

Week 2

▪ DAY 8

Breakfast: Avocado-Cucumber Soup

Lunch: Quinoa Detox Bowl

Dinner: Lemon-Cilantro Cauliflower Rice + Steamed Broccoli

Snack: Cucumber-Mint Detox Water

▪ DAY 9

Breakfast: Detox Apple Chia Bowl

Lunch: Zucchini Noodles with Pesto

Dinner: Roasted Beet & Garlic Soup + Kale Chips (Immune recipe)

Snack: Mold-Free Coconut Yogurt Parfait

▪ DAY 10

Breakfast: Turmeric-Almond Milk Tonic

Lunch: Cabbage Slaw + Avocado slices

Dinner: Baked Wild Cod with Parsley + Lemon-Carrot Purée (Kidney recipe)

Snack: Alkaline Seed Crackers

▪ DAY 11

Breakfast: Alkaline Green Juice

Lunch: Lentil & Kale Stew

Dinner: Quinoa Detox Bowl + Mold-Free Stir-Fry

Snack: Ginger-Lime Marinated Mushrooms

DAY 12

Breakfast: Mold-Free Coconut Yogurt Parfait
Lunch: Fennel & Arugula Salad
Dinner: Garlic-Ginger Salmon + Lemon Carrots
Snack: Avocado-Cucumber Soup

DAY 13

Breakfast: Turmeric-Almond Milk Tonic
Lunch: Zucchini Noodles with Pesto
Dinner: Spaghetti Squash with Basil Sauce
Snack: Cucumber-Mint Detox Water

DAY 14

Breakfast: Avocado-Cucumber Soup
Lunch: Roasted Veggies + Kale & Quinoa Bowl
Dinner: Mold-Free Alkaline Veggie Stir-Fry
Snack: Ginger-Lime Mushrooms

Week 3

DAY 15

Breakfast: Detox Apple Chia Bowl
Lunch: Cabbage Detox Soup
Dinner: Lemon-Cilantro Cauliflower Rice + Wild Cod
Snack: Mold-Free Coconut Yogurt Parfait

📓 DAY 16

Breakfast: Alkaline Green Juice
Lunch: Quinoa Detox Bowl
Dinner: Steamed Broccoli + Baked Salmon
Snack: Fennel Salad

📓 DAY 17

Breakfast: Avocado-Cucumber Soup
Lunch: Warm Kale & Quinoa Salad
Dinner: Garlic Soup + Lemon Carrots
Snack: Alkaline Seed Crackers

📓 DAY 18

Breakfast: Turmeric-Almond Milk Tonic
Lunch: Zucchini Noodles with Pesto
Dinner: Mold-Free Stir-Fry + Beet Salad
Snack: Cucumber-Mint Detox Water

📓 DAY 19

Breakfast: Mold-Free Coconut Yogurt Parfait
Lunch: Spaghetti Squash with Garlic-Basil Sauce
Dinner: Cabbage Soup + Broccoli with Garlic Oil
Snack: Ginger-Lime Mushrooms

DAY 20

Breakfast: Alkaline Green Juice
Lunch: Fennel & Arugula Salad
Dinner: Baked Cod + Cauliflower Rice
Snack: Turmeric Almond Milk

DAY 21

Breakfast: Detox Apple Chia Bowl
Lunch: Quinoa Detox Bowl
Dinner: Steamed Veggie Platter + Pesto Dip
Snack: Mold-Free Coconut Yogurt Parfait

Week 4

DAY 22

Breakfast: Chilled Avocado and Cucumber Soup

Lunch: Zucchini Noodles with Herbal Pesto

Dinner: Wild-Caught Cod with Lemon-Glazed Carrots

Snack: Mushrooms Marinated in Ginger and Lime

DAY 23

Breakfast: Warm Turmeric and Almond Milk Elixir

Lunch: Hearty Lentil and Kale Stew

Dinner: Mold-Free Vegetable Stir-Fry with Cauliflower Rice

Snack: Mineral-Rich Alkaline Seed Crackers

DAY 24

Breakfast: Mold-Free Coconut Yogurt Parfait

Lunch: Roasted Beet Soup

Dinner: Spaghetti Squash + Lemon Broccoli

Snack: Cucumber-Mint Detox Water

DAY 25

Breakfast: Alkaline Green Juice

Lunch: Fennel & Arugula Salad

Dinner: Cabbage Soup + Carrots

Snack: Ginger-Lime Mushrooms

DAY 26

Breakfast: Avocado-Cucumber Soup

Lunch: Warm Kale & Quinoa Bowl

Dinner: Mold-Free Stir-Fry + Lemon-Cilantro Cauliflower Rice

Snack: Mold-Free Coconut Yogurt Parfait

DAY 27

Breakfast: Detox Apple Chia Bowl

Lunch: Zucchini Noodles with Pesto

Dinner: Baked Wild Cod + Broccoli

Snack: Cucumber-Mint Detox Water

DAY 28

Breakfast: Turmeric-Almond Milk Tonic

Lunch: Cabbage Slaw + Kale Chips

Dinner: Garlic Soup + Quinoa

Snack: Ginger-Lime Mushrooms

DAY 29

Breakfast: Mold-Free Coconut Yogurt Parfait

Lunch: Fennel Salad + Detox Broth

Dinner: Spaghetti Squash with Garlic Sauce

Snack: Alkaline Seed Crackers

DAY 30

Breakfast: Alkaline Green Juice

Lunch: Lentil Stew + Kale

Dinner: Mold-Free Stir-Fry + Beet & Quinoa Bowl

Snack: Turmeric Almond Milk

Conclusion: Returning to Nature, Reclaiming Your Health

As we close the final chapter of **THE CURE FOR ALL DISEASES COOKBOOK**, we return to the foundation on which this entire work was built: the belief that the human body was designed to heal itself when given the right tools and freed from interference. These tools—clean food, medicinal herbs, non-toxic environments, and a connection to the rhythms of nature—are ancient, powerful, and, most importantly, accessible to all.

Throughout this book, we've journeyed through the core principles of Dr. Hulda Regehr Clark's work: the role of parasites, toxins, **and pollutants in disease formation;** the importance of detoxifying the liver, **kidneys, and digestive system;** and the utility of natural therapies including herbs, frequency-based tools like the zapper, and, of course, food as a primary form of medicine.

But this cookbook has not only presented theory—it has been a practical companion. **With over 75 recipes and a full 30-day healing meal plan,** this work was crafted to support your transformation from illness, stagnation, or fatigue toward vibrant, sustainable wellness.

Let us now reflect on the key messages and offer some guidance as you continue this path forward.

Healing Is Simpler Than We've Been Told

Conventional medicine frequently functions within a framework of complexity. We are taught that disease is the result of mysterious genetics or random chance. Yet what Dr. Clark unveiled—and what many other pioneers in natural health have echoed—is that much of human illness is not mysterious at all. It is logical, cause-and-effect. Parasites, heavy metals, mold, solvents, industrial chemicals, and dietary poisons are not just abstract concerns; they are real and measurable invaders that impair the function of organs, confuse the immune system, and disrupt cellular harmony.

When these root causes are identified and removed—and when the organs of detoxification are supported with herbal protocols, natural foods, and healing frequencies—the body often returns to balance with a grace that may seem miraculous, but is in truth simply nature restored.

This is not wishful thinking or placebo. It is biology.

Food Is a Biological Language

Food is not just fuel. It is information. Every bite you take sends a message to your cells—messages that can inflame or calm, energize or exhaust, nourish or burden.

In this cookbook, we've offered you foods that send the right messages—meals that whisper to your immune system, "**Stand strong**"; that sing to your liver, "**Detoxify freely**"; that remind your microbiome,

"**Flourish and protect.**" These meals are more than delicious—they are biologically intelligent.

The recipes have been crafted to be free from mold-promoting ingredients, allergenic additives, and processed toxins. They favor whole, alkaline, organic produce, herbs with antiparasitic and anti-inflammatory properties, and simple combinations that reduce digestive stress.

When you eat this way consistently, your body doesn't have to fight your food—it uses it to heal.

The Kitchen Is Your Pharmacy

This book reclaims the idea that healing doesn't have to come from a pill bottle or a sterile clinic. True healing begins at home, particularly in your kitchen.

Each time you chop garlic, steep dandelion root tea, or prepare a detoxifying broth, you are practicing a form of medicine that predates pharmaceuticals by millennia. You become both chef and healer—an active participant in your wellness rather than a passive recipient of treatments.

Herbs like black walnut hull, wormwood, turmeric, and milk thistle were featured not just because they're trendy, but because their healing properties have been documented in folk medicine, scientific literature, and clinical observation. By incorporating these into your diet, you aren't just eating—you're cleansing.

The Zapper and Frequency Medicine

While this is a cookbook, it would be incomplete without honoring Dr. Clark's unique contributions to frequency-based healing. Her discovery that every pathogen emits a distinct frequency—and that these can be disrupted using a simple homemade electronic device—radically changed how we understand disease.

The zapper, as she called it, is not meant to replace good nutrition or herbal cleansing. Rather, it works in harmony with them. As you clear your body of toxins through food, the zapper can assist by weakening or eliminating the microorganisms that no longer have a supportive terrain in which to thrive.

You now know how to build and use this tool—and you understand its role in the broader system of natural healing. Paired with the right food, it becomes even more effective.

What to Expect As You Heal

Healing is rarely linear. As you detox, you may experience symptoms of cleansing: fatigue, mild headaches, rashes, or changes in bowel function. This is the body's way of flushing out years—sometimes decades—of accumulated waste.

Be gentle with yourself. Stay hydrated. Rest deeply. Listen to your body's signals.

And most importantly, persist.

True healing does not come in a bottle. It comes from commitment. The more you support your body, the more resilient and radiant you become.

A Final Word: Empowerment

This cookbook was never meant to make you dependent on it—or on any one system. It was meant to empower you. To wake you up to the truth that the body you inhabit is intelligent, adaptive, and wise beyond modern comprehension.

It doesn't need synthetic drugs for every ache or surgery for every dysfunction. It needs clarity, clean inputs, and unburdening. It needs food that honors nature.

You now have tools, recipes, protocols, and frameworks to move forward. You've built a parasite-free pantry. You've nourished your liver and kidneys. You've supported detoxification and alkalinity. You've reduced the burden of mold, metals, and inflammation.

What you do next is up to you.

Will you return to the convenience foods, the microwave dinners, the toxic oils, and mold-ridden grains? Or will you continue on the path of wisdom—of garlic, greens, roots, and broths?

The decision is yours, but the reward is universal: a life of vitality, clarity, and freedom from unnecessary suffering.

You don't need to fear disease when you understand its origins. You don't need to rely on experts when you understand your body. And you don't need to wait for permission to heal.

You are your own healer. Your kitchen is your apothecary. Your food is your cure.

May this book serve not just as a guide, **but as a catalyst—a spark that reignites your belief in the ancient truth:**

Healing begins with what's on your plate, and health is your birthright.

To your continued wellness

Printed in Dunstable, United Kingdom

67930176R00067